This book is a collection of medicinal herbal tea recipes Rose has passed down to her children and grandchildren.

In a large heat resistant glass pitcher, she adds two tea bags and then the fresh herbs she needs for the day.

You can drink this pot of tea throughout the day either hot, room temperture or on ice.

Note: Extremely large doses of herbs or consuming for a prolonged period of time may trigger serious side effects.

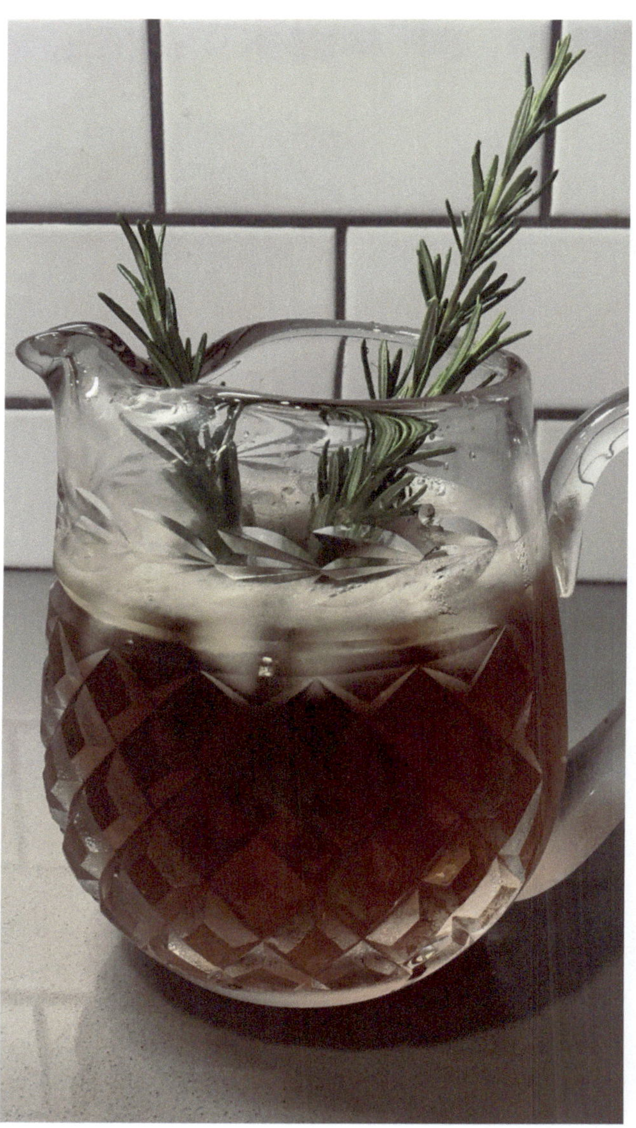

Tea Recipes

For a small pitcher use one tea bag and for a large pitcher use two. For each recipe use all or any of the suggested herbs and a wedge of seasonal fruit.

Cold or Flu
Any herbal fruit tea,
add oregano, thyme, elderberry,
sage and ginger

Sleep
Chamomile tea with lavender

Upset Stomach
Green or black tea, add mint, chamomile
and fennel

Cramps
Any herbal tea, add fennel, ginger
and lemon balm

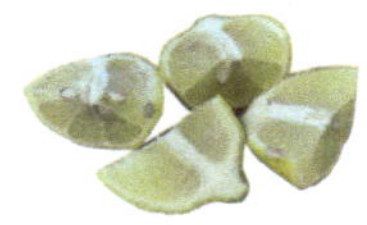

Tea Recipes

Fever
Green tea, add linden pods.
This tea will sweat out a fever.

Inflamation
Green tea, add rosemary, cloves,
cinnamon and ginger

Headaches
Black or green tea, add peppermint,
ginger, rosemary, linden pods
and feverfew

Depression & Anxiety
Green tea add, lavender, chamomile,
lemon balm and St. John's wort

Purify Blood
Herbal fruit tea, add dandelion and nettle

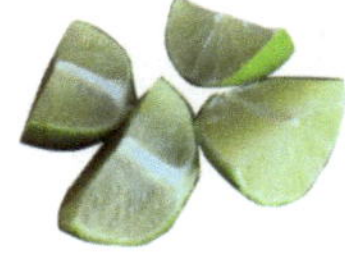

Tea Recipes

Bladder Infections
Green tea, Uva Ursi and cranberry juice

Special Brews

Congestion
Fill a saucepan with water. Add thyme and
sage bring to a boil. Cover your head
with a towel and inhale the steam.

Pink Eye and Eye Infections
Boil water and add chamomile, let it seep.
Soak cotton balls in mixture and
use as a warm compress.

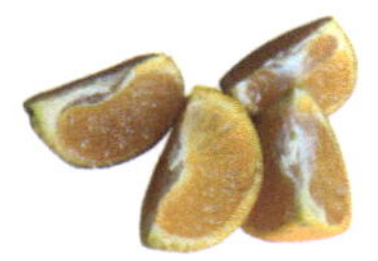

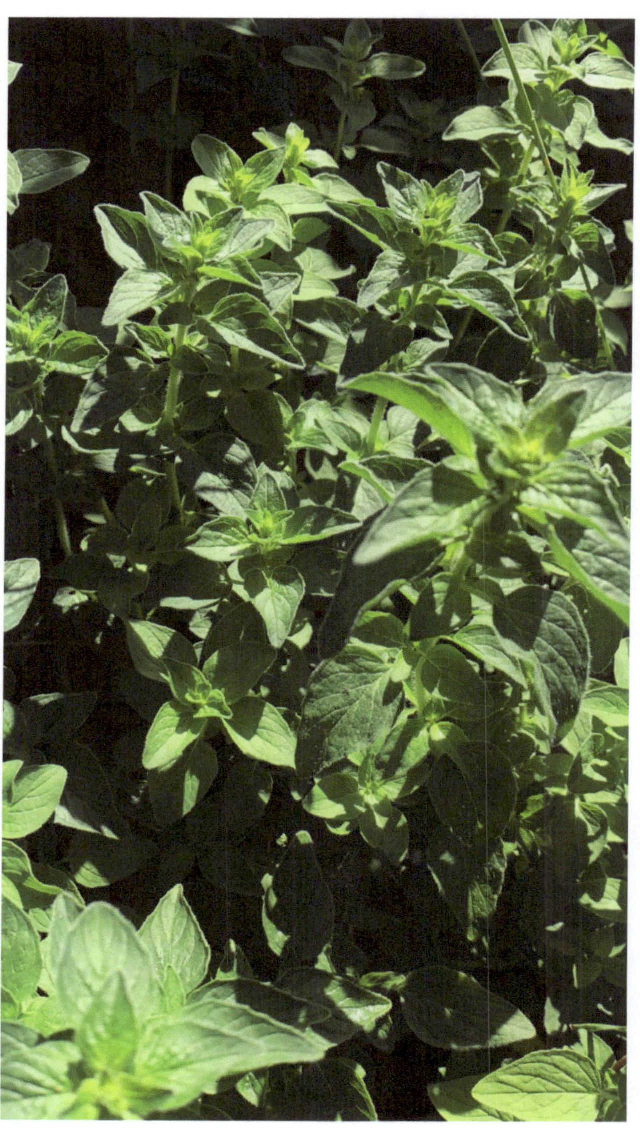

Oregano

Tea Use
Add Oregano leaves to boost the immune system and to help fight off colds and flu.

Medicinal Uses
Topical pain relief, such as
with a toothache.

Oregano oil in a diffuser or vaporizer
may help to alleviate sinus and chest
congestion, and reduce cough symptoms.

Antifungal and antiviral properties.
Oregano oil can be applied to the skin for
conditions like acne, cold sores and
dandruff, and for the relief
of sore, aching muscles and joints.

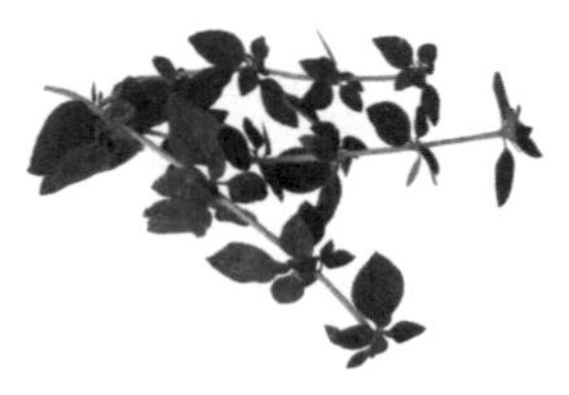

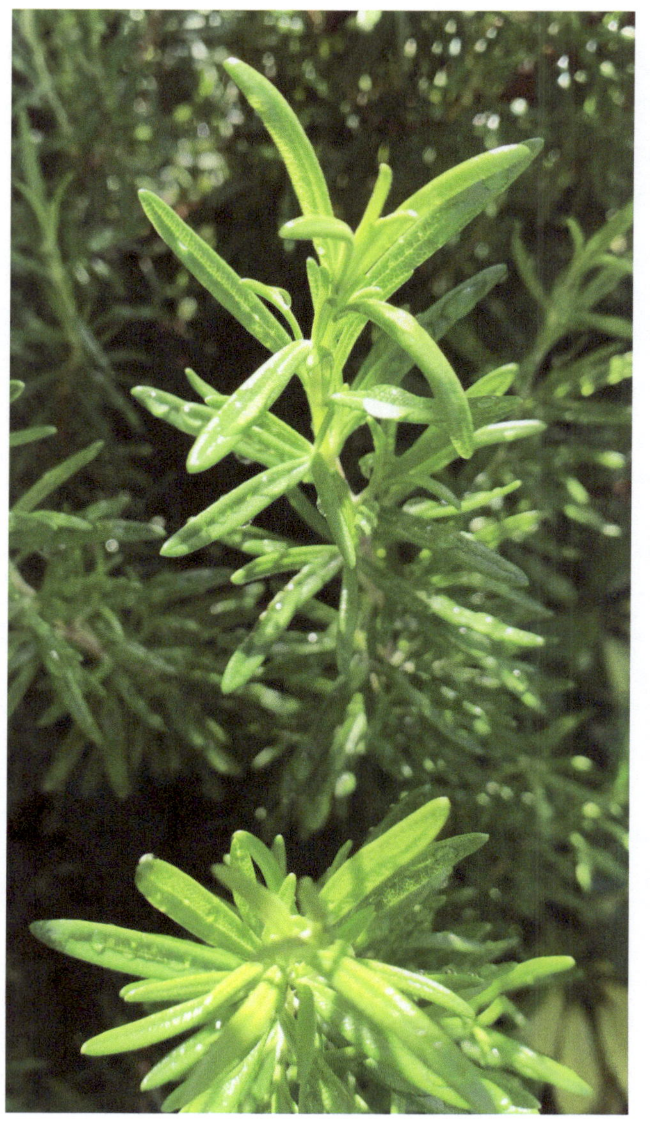

Rosemary

Tea Use
Add Rosemary leaves to help
reduce inflamation, reduce headache and
boost the immune and circulatory system.

Medicinal Use
Alleviate Muscle Pain
Improves Memory
Boost Circulate System
Promotes Hair Growth

Burn Rosemary to disinfect rooms
and eliminate germs.

Fun Fact
Rosemary is a symbol of loyalty and love.
In certain parts of the world, bride, groom
and their guests wear branches of
rosemary during wedding ceremonies.

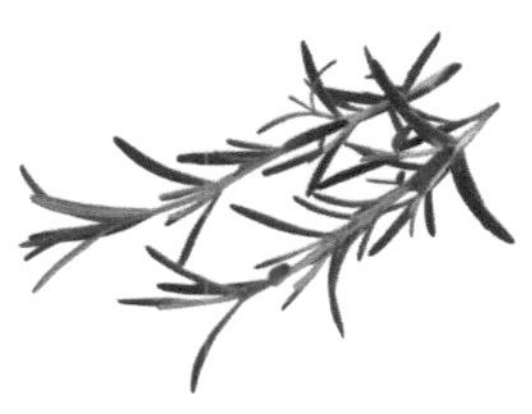

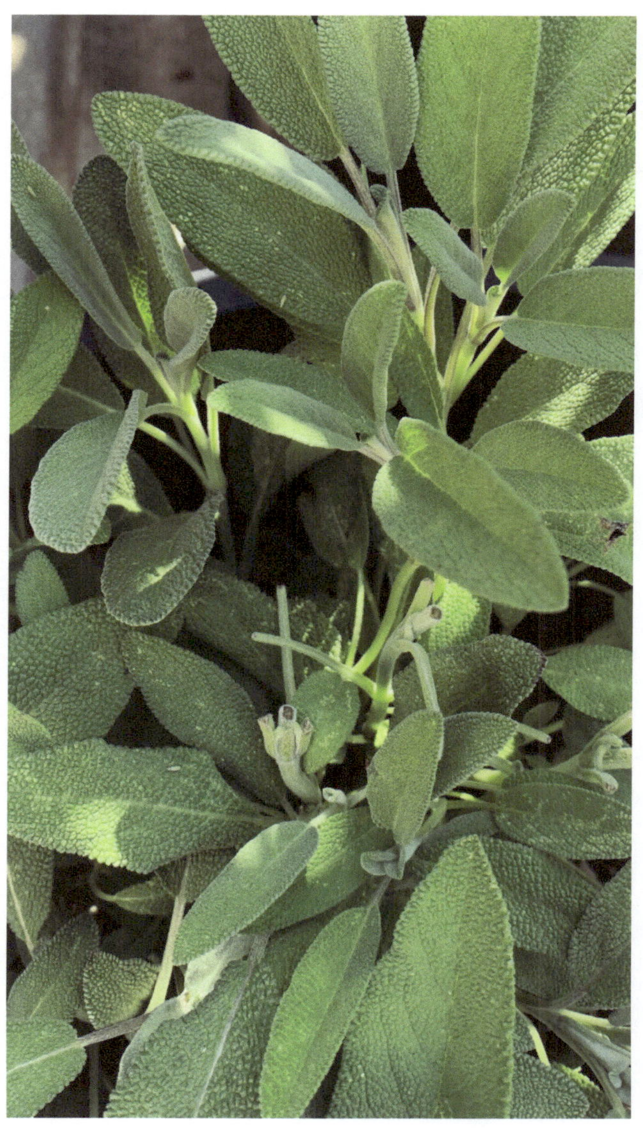

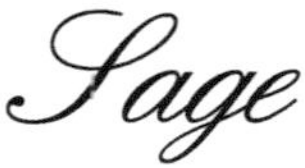

Sage

Tea Use
Add Sage leaves to treat colds, coughs, digestion and circulation problems.

Medicinal Use
Topical uses are antibacterial, antiseptic, anti-inflamtory, astringent, and antiviral.

Burn Sage smudge stick to purify the air.

Fun Fact
The Greeks were the first to cultivate Sage. The Romans considered it a sacred plant and gathering Sage was a ceremonious affair.

Too much Sage can make you agitated.

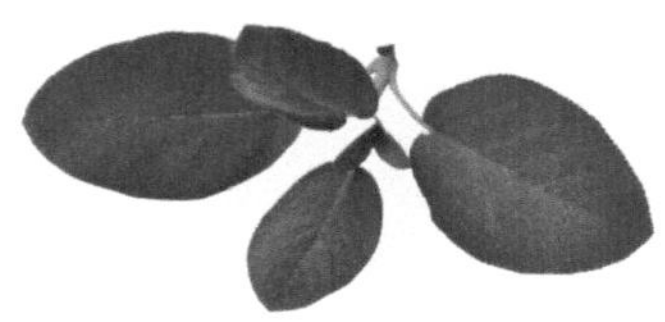

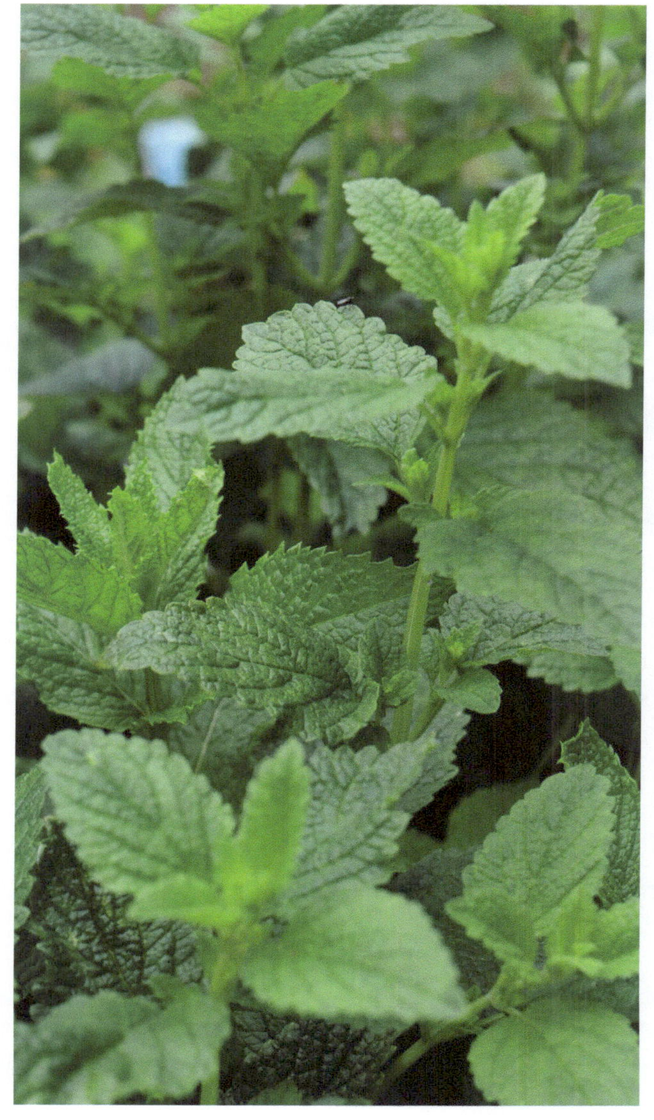

Mint

Tea use
Add mint leaves to calm your stomach.

Medicinal Use
Stimulates Digestive Enzymes
Alleviates Indigestion
Gas and Cramps
Anti-inflammatory
May aid in weigh loss.

Fun Fact
Mint gets its name from *Menthe* a
Greek mythical character. Ancient Romans
and Greeks used mint to flavor
cordials and fruit compotes, also for baths
and perfumes.

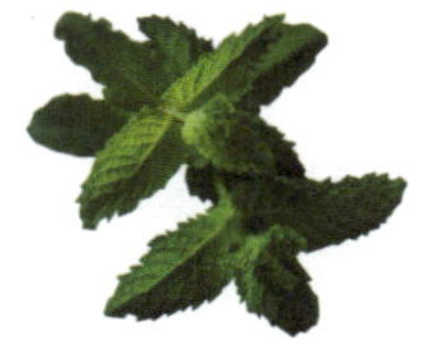

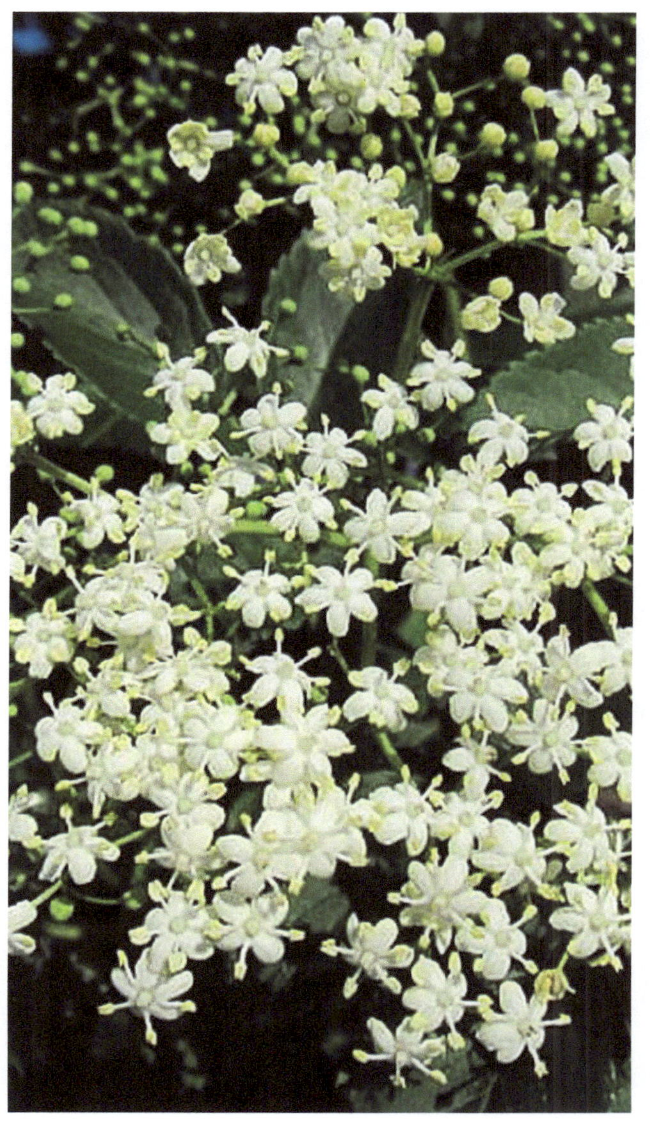

Elderberry

Tea Use
Add to shorten the lengh of a cold.
Both the berries and flowers boost the
immune system.

Medicinal Use
Reduces symptoms of sinusitis
and bronchitis.
Back & Leg Pain
Nerve Pain
Chronic fatique Syndrome

Fun Fact
Crushed elderberry leaves release an
unpleasant smell. In the past people
used these leaves, attached to the
horse's mane, to repel flies.

Note: Stems are poisonious

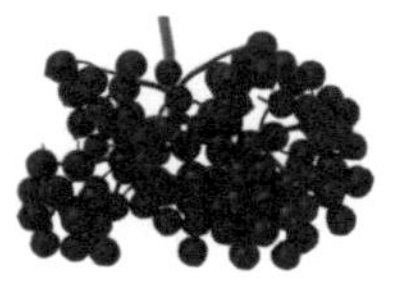

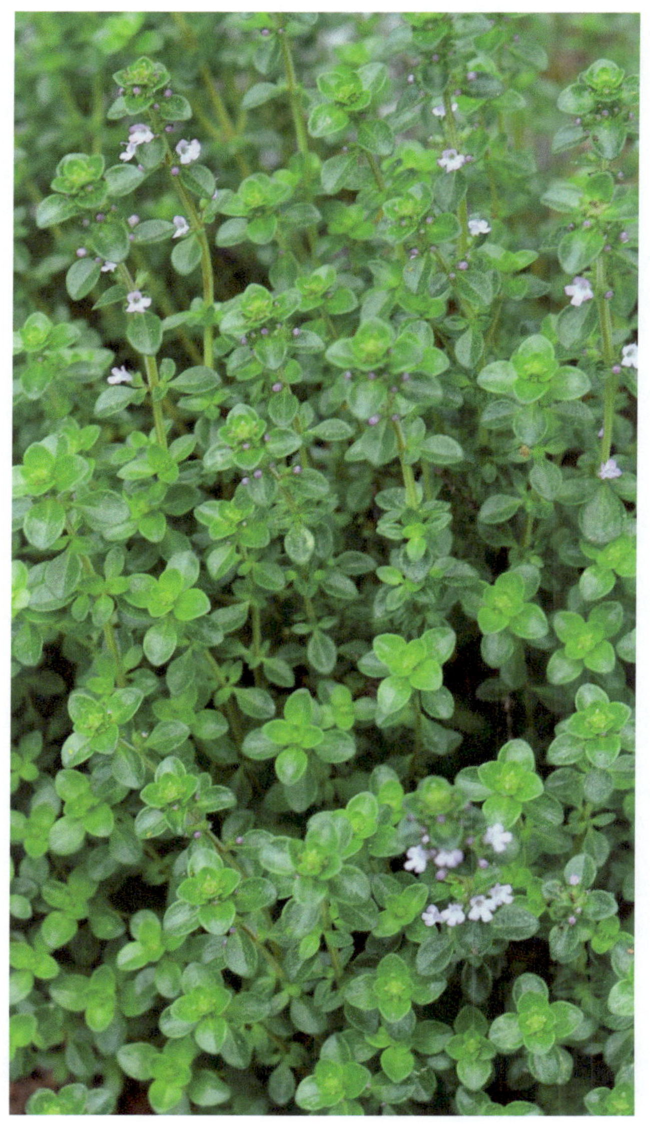

Thyme

Tea Use
Add Thyme leaves when you have
bronchitis or sore throat.

Medicinal Use
Colic
Arthritis
Upset Stomach
Diarrhea
Intestinal Gas
Parasitic Worm Infections
Skin Disorders
Antiseptic

Fun Fact
The Ancient Greeks considered thyme
to be a source of courage.

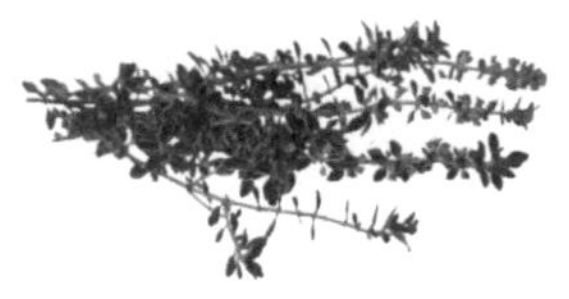

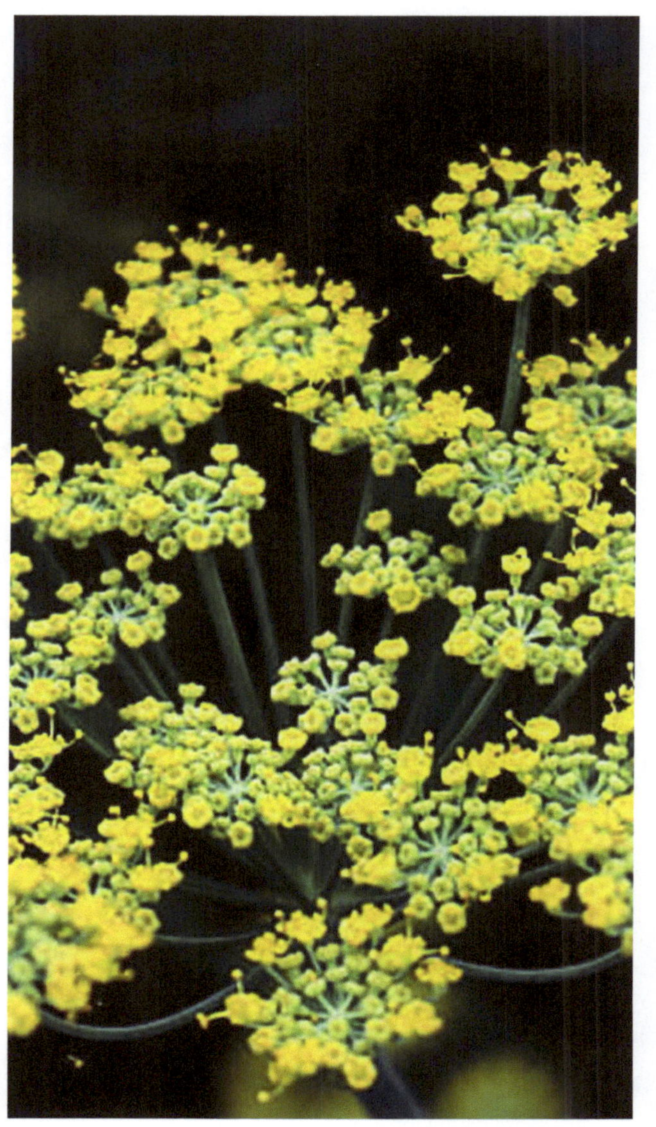

Fennel

Tea Use
Add the flowers, leaves or seeds
for a digestive aid. It reduces digestive
cramping, gas and bloating.

Medicinal Use
The leaves are full of phytochemicals.
Folklore says these may reduce or block
the growth of cancer cells and suppress
the developement of tumours.

Fun Fact
According to Greek mythology,
Prometheus stole fire from the Gods and
gave it as a gift to mankind.
It was the stalk of a fennel plant that he
used to steal the fire!

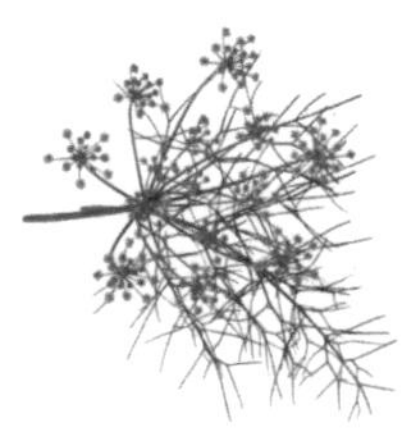

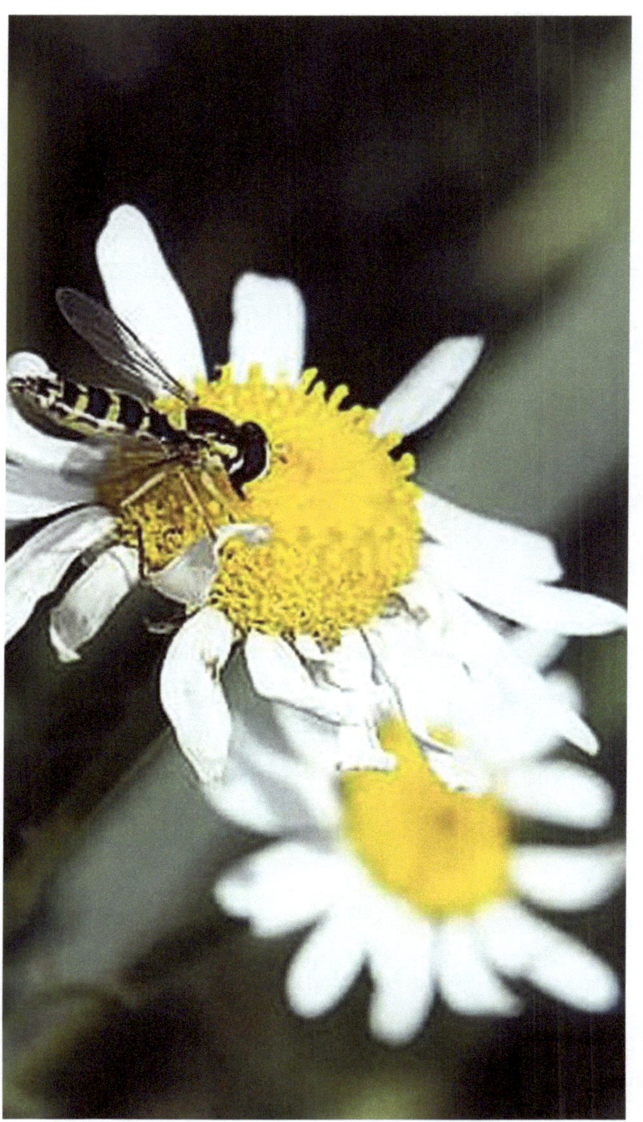

Chamomile

Tea Use
Add chamomile flowers to calm an
upset stomach, help you sleep, calm
anxiety
and aid in digestion.

Medicinal Use
Remedy for Pink Eye
Healing Salve
Reduces Toothache

Fun Fact
Chamomile was used in the process of
mummification in ancient Egypt.

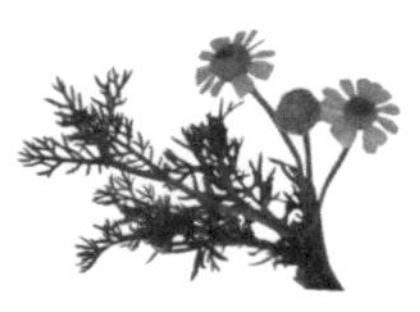

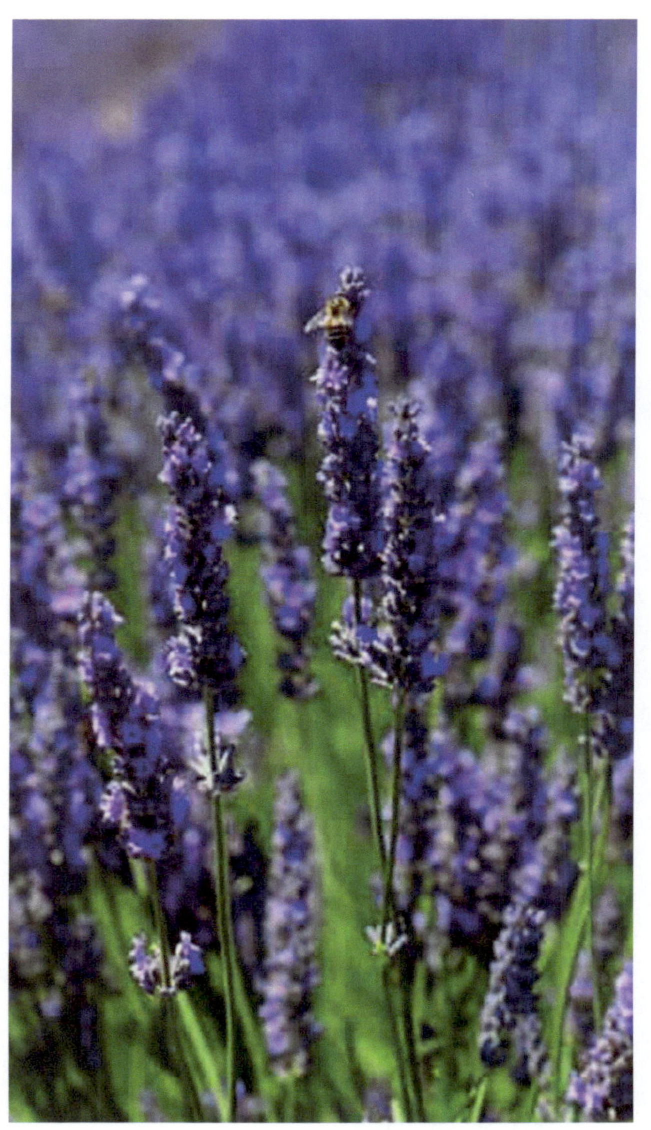

Lavender

Tea Use
Add either flowers or leaves or both for
anxiety, insominia, restlessness

Medicinal Use
Anti-inflammatory
Antiseptic
Minor Burns
Bug Bites

Fun Fact
During the Bubonic Plague in the
17th century, lavender was used as a
remedy to ward off potential disease.

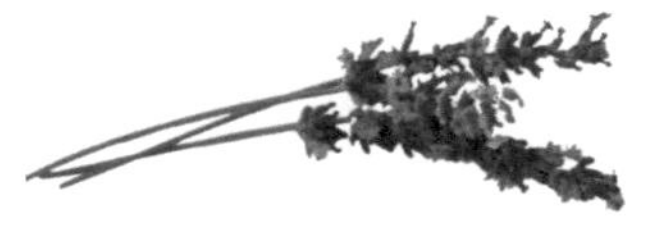

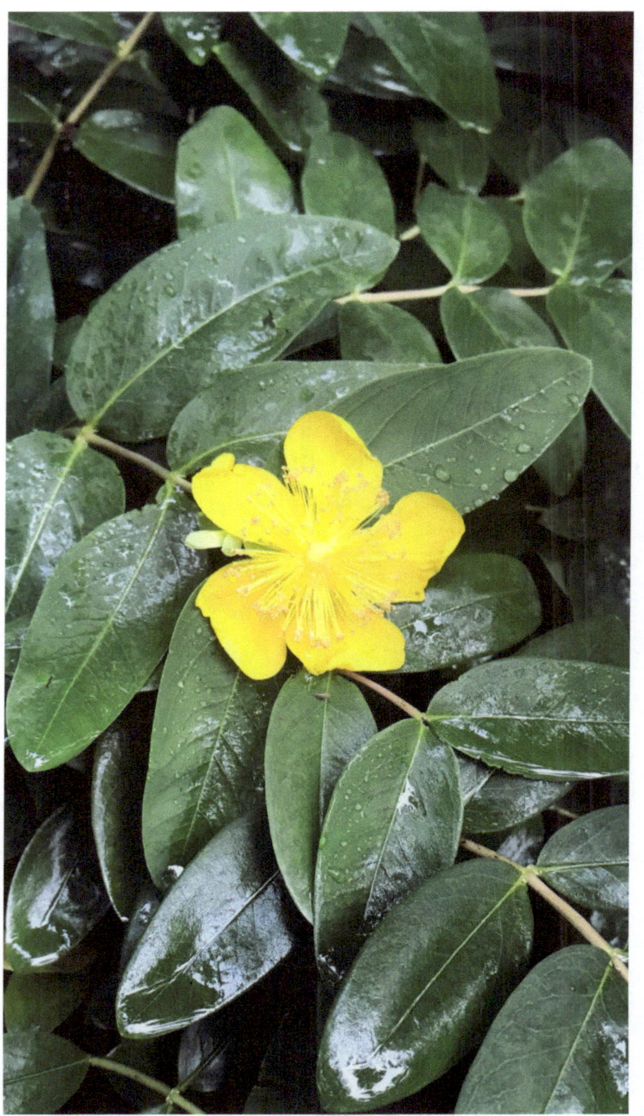

St John's Wort

Tea Use
Add fresh flowers for depressive disorders or low mood. It helps by increasing serotonin.The flowering tops of the St. John's wort plant are used to prepare teas.

Not So Fun Fact
When the petals of the yellow St. John's wort flowers are rubbed together, a resin is released, leaving a red stain. Legend says that this is because the plant sprung up from the blood of John the Baptist when he was beheaded.

Note: St. John's wort can cause serious interactions with some medications.

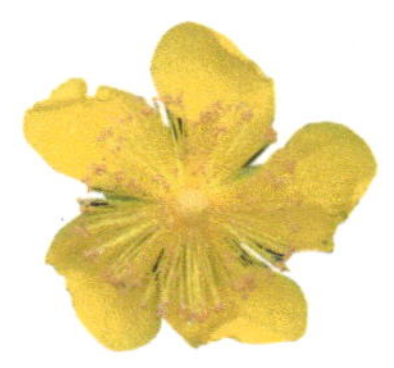

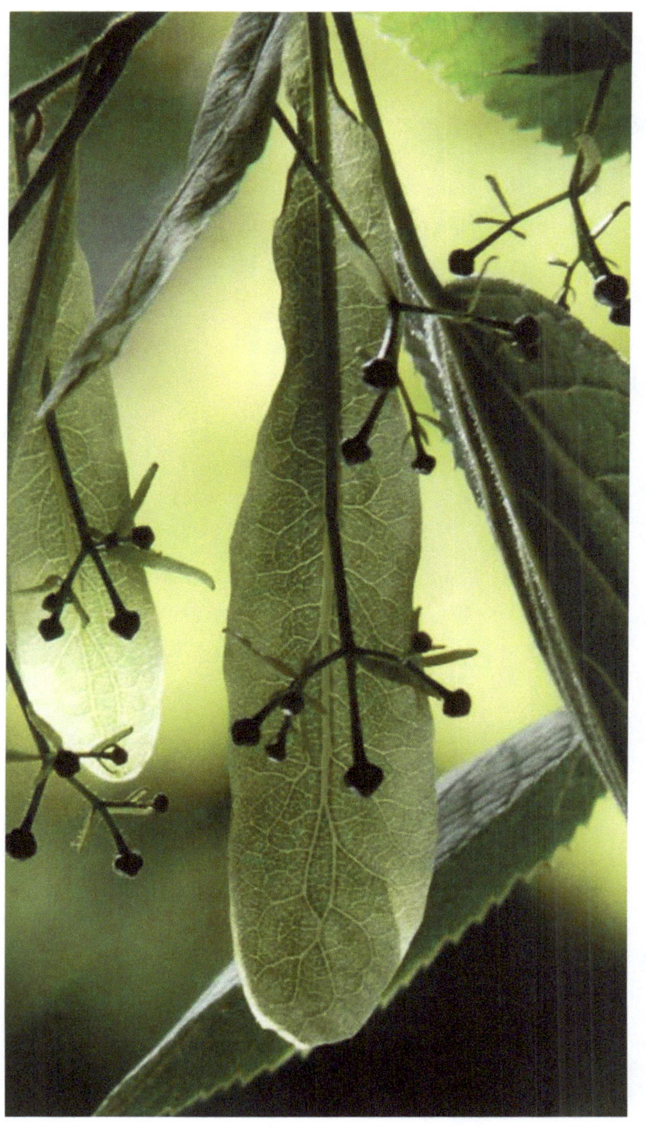

Linden

Tea Use
Add the Linden tree pods to sweat out a
fever from a cold, flu or infection.

Medicinal Use
Nasal Congestion
Relieve Throat Irritation
Add to a lotion to reduce itchy skin.

Fun Fact
The Linden tree usually has a lifespan of
a few hundred years, but there are
specimens thought to be more than
1,000 years old.

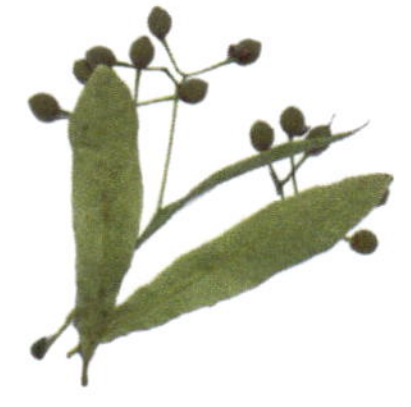

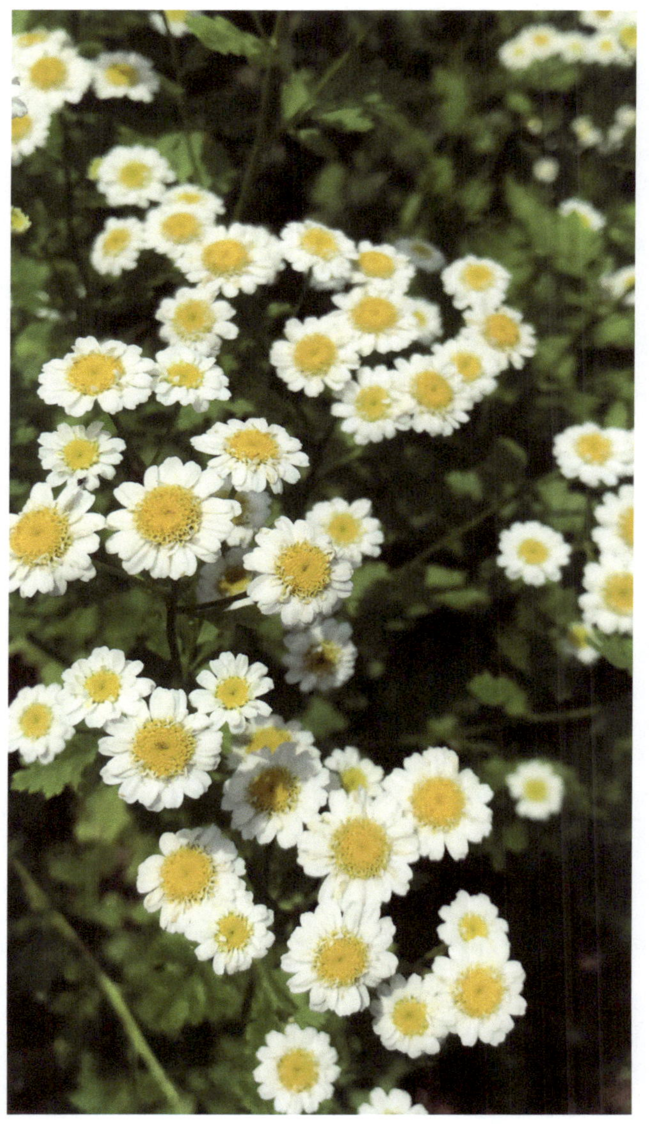

Feverfew

Tea Use
Add Feverfew leaves to bring down a fever or help with migraines.

Medicinal Use
Rheumatoid Arthritis
Stomach Aches
Toothaches
Insect Bites
Infertility and problems
with menstruation

Fun Fact
The name stems from the Latin word *febrifugia*, "fever reducer." The first century Greek physician, Dioscorides, prescribed feverfew for all hot inflammations.

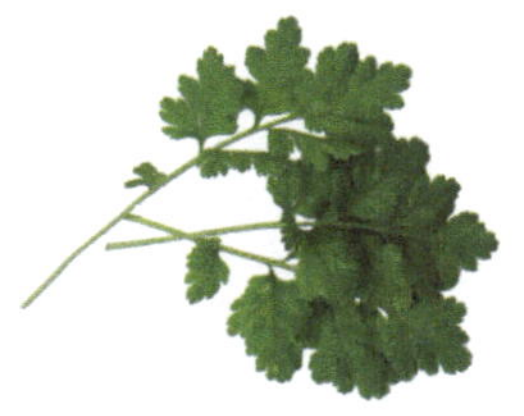

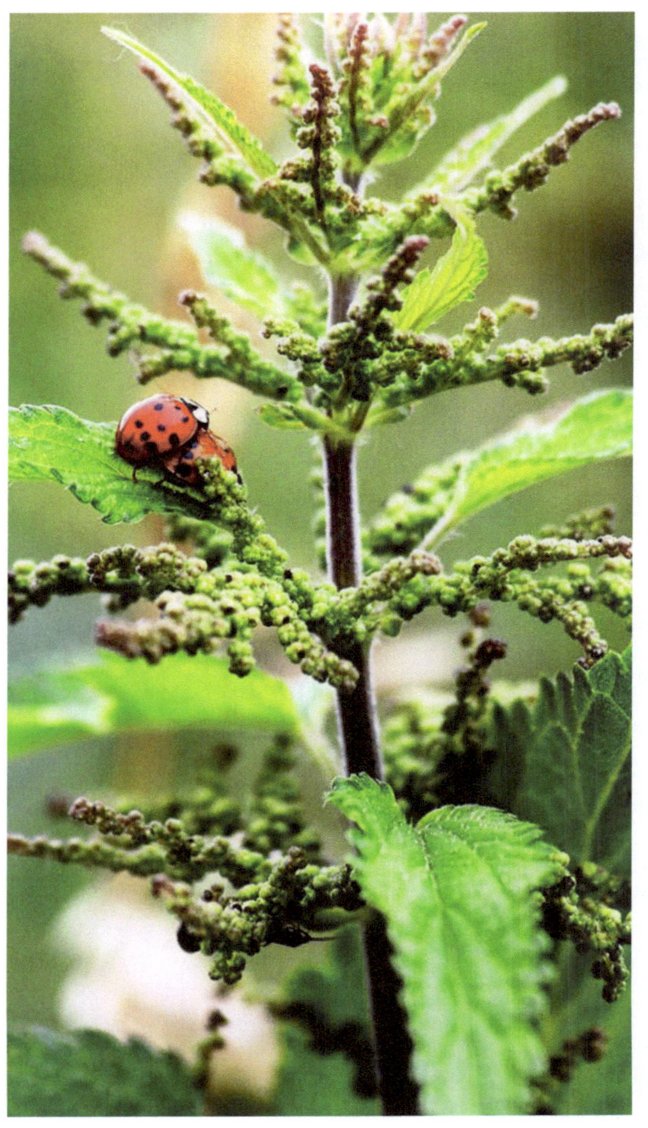

Nettle

Tea Use
Add Nettle leaves for urinary problems
and
to purify blood.

Medicinal Use
Painful Muscles & Joints
Eczema
Arthritis
Anemia

Fun Fact
Full of vitamins A, C and some B vitamins.
Fresh nettles also contain potassium,
calcium, chromium, copper, magnesium,
and iron.
Nettles sting to prevent them from
being eaten by animals.

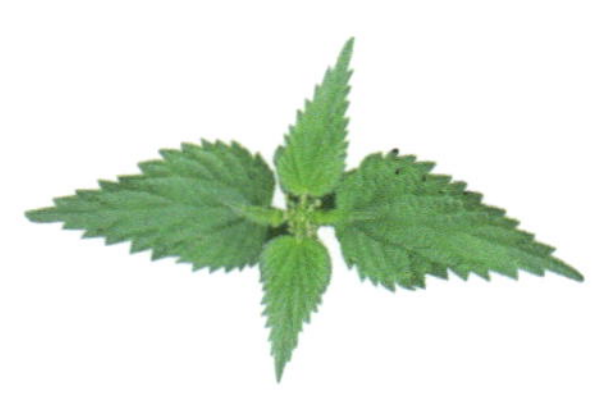

Notes

Notes

Notes

Notes

PRAYER

Herr gieb mir helle
Augen die Schönheit der Welt zu sehn.

Herr gieb mir feine Ohren
Dein Rufen zu versteh und weiche
liebe Hände fur unser
Brüder Leid und klingende
Worte für diese wirre Zeit.

Translation:

*Lord please give me bright eyes
to see the beauty of this world.*

*Lord please give me open ears
to hear your calling and give me gentle
hands for the suffering of the sick and
good words for this troubled world.*